LOW POTASSIUM DIET

A Comprehensive Guide to Managing Your Health

Adams .U. Morris

TABLE OF CONTENTS

CHAPTER 1

Introduction to Low Potassium Diet

In our fast-paced world, we often don't think much about the nutrients our bodies need to function optimally. Potassium, however, is a critical mineral that plays a significant role in our overall health, and understanding its importance is the first step towards a successful low potassium diet.

The Basics of Potassium: Potassium is a mineral and an

electrolyte, a term that might sound complex but is essential to comprehend when discussing a low potassium diet. Electrolytes are electrically charged minerals that help balance fluid levels in our bodies, maintain proper muscle function, and ensure our nerves function correctly. Potassium is one of the key electrolytes, and it excels at helping muscles contract, including our most vital muscle, the heart.

The Role of Potassium: Potassium is involved in countless bodily processes. It's crucial for maintaining normal blood pressure, as it helps to relax the walls of blood vessels, making it easier for the heart to pump blood. Without adequate potassium, blood pressure can rise, potentially leading to cardiovascular issues.

Furthermore, potassium is essential for proper muscle function, from the muscles used for lifting weights to the involuntary muscles that control digestion and breathing. It helps regulate nerve impulses, allowing our brains to communicate effectively with the rest of the body.

Why Low Potassium Diets Are Necessary: Now that we understand the importance of potassium, you might wonder why anyone would need a low potassium diet. The answer lies in specific medical conditions, the most common being kidney disease.

When our kidneys are healthy, they filter excess potassium from our blood and excrete it through urine. However, in kidney disease, the kidneys lose this ability. High levels of potassium can build up in the bloodstream, leading to a condition called hyperkalemia. This condition can cause irregular heart rhythms, muscle weakness, and even heart attacks in severe cases. Hence, individuals with kidney disease, especially those on dialysis, are often advised to follow a low potassium diet.

Other medical conditions may also necessitate a low potassium diet. These can include certain heart conditions and medications that increase potassium levels in the blood. In such cases, a low potassium diet can help manage these conditions and reduce the risk of complications.

Understanding Low Potassium Foods: Before we dive into the specifics of a low potassium diet, it's crucial to understand what foods are high in potassium. Potassium-rich foods include bananas, oranges, potatoes, tomatoes, and various leafy greens. These foods are not inherently unhealthy; in fact, they offer a wealth of vitamins and minerals. However, for individuals who need to restrict their potassium intake, these foods must be consumed in moderation or replaced with lower-potassium alternatives.

The Importance of Reading Food Labels: To effectively manage a low potassium diet, you'll become intimately familiar with food labels. Food manufacturers are required to list the potassium content of their products on nutrition labels. This information is a lifeline for anyone on a low potassium diet.

When reading labels, pay close attention to the "potassium" or "K" value. Foods containing 200 milligrams (mg) or more of potassium per serving are generally considered high-potassium foods. It's essential to track your daily potassium intake and stay within the limits recommended by your healthcare provider.

The Impact of Cooking Methods: Cooking can significantly influence the potassium content of foods. For instance, boiling vegetables can leach potassium into the cooking water, making the vegetables themselves lower in potassium. Therefore, it's important to be mindful of how you prepare your meals.

Steaming, microwaving, and roasting are cooking methods that help retain the potassium content of foods. Additionally, you can reduce potassium content by choosing specific cuts of meat and trimming away excess fat, as potassium tends to accumulate in animal tissues.

In summary, this chapter has laid the foundation for understanding the importance of potassium, its role in the body, and why some individuals need to follow a low potassium diet. We've also touched on the significance of reading food labels and the impact of cooking methods on potassium content. Armed with this knowledge, you're now ready to embark on your journey to a healthier life through a low potassium diet. The subsequent chapters will provide you with more in-depth information on how to make this dietary adjustment successfully, tailored to your specific needs.

CHAPTER 2

Understanding Potassium Sources

Now that we've established the importance of potassium and why some individuals may need to follow a low potassium diet, it's time to delve deeper into the world of potassium sources. This chapter will be your guide to identifying foods high in potassium, deciphering nutrition labels, and understanding how various cooking methods can impact potassium content.

Potassium-Rich Foods:

Potassium is naturally present in a wide range of foods, and recognizing these sources is fundamental when you're on a low potassium diet. Here are some common foods that are typically high in potassium:

1. **Bananas:** Bananas are often the poster child for potassium-rich foods. A medium-sized banana contains around 400-450 milligrams of potassium.

2. **Oranges and Orange Juice:** Citrus fruits like oranges and their juices are

potassium-rich. A cup of orange juice can contain approximately 500 milligrams of potassium.

3. **Potatoes:** Whether they're mashed, baked, or fried, potatoes are a significant source of potassium. A medium-sized potato can provide around 900 milligrams of potassium.

4. **Tomatoes and Tomato Products:** Tomatoes and tomato-based products like sauces and soups are potassium-packed. A cup of tomato sauce can contain

900 milligrams of potassium.

5. **Leafy Greens:** Vegetables like spinach, kale, and Swiss chard are nutrient powerhouses but can also be high in potassium. A cup of cooked spinach may contain over 800 milligrams of potassium.

6. **Avocado:** Avocado is a unique fruit as it's high in healthy fats and potassium. A medium-sized avocado can contain around 700 milligrams of potassium.

7. **Dried Fruits:** Dried fruits like raisins, apricots, and

prunes are concentrated sources of potassium. A small box of raisins can provide about 600 milligrams of potassium.

8. **Beans and Legumes:** Foods like kidney beans, black beans, and lentils are excellent sources of plant-based protein but also contain a fair amount of potassium. A cup of cooked kidney beans can contain approximately 700 milligrams of potassium.

9. **Fish:** Certain types of fish, such as salmon and tuna, can be relatively high in

potassium. A 3-ounce serving of cooked salmon can provide about 450 milligrams of potassium.

10. **Nuts and Seeds:** While nuts and seeds are nutritious, they can also contribute to your potassium intake. For example, an ounce of almonds may contain around 200 milligrams of potassium.

Understanding these common sources of potassium is crucial when you're following a low potassium diet. However, it's essential to note that not all individuals need to avoid all of these foods entirely. The severity of potassium restriction depends on your specific medical condition and the guidance of your healthcare provider.

Deciphering Food Labels:

In today's world, where pre-packaged and processed foods are prevalent, understanding how to read food labels is a vital skill for anyone on a low potassium diet. Here's a breakdown of what to look for on food labels:

1. **Potassium Content:** Check the nutrition label for

the "Potassium" or "K" value. Foods containing 200 milligrams (mg) or more of potassium per serving are generally considered high-potassium foods.

2. **Serving Size:** Pay attention to the serving size listed on the label. Your potassium intake depends on the size of the portion you consume. Sometimes, a small serving size may have acceptable potassium levels, even if the overall content in the entire package is high.

3. **% Daily Value (%DV):** The %DV indicates how

much a nutrient in a serving of food contributes to a daily diet. It's usually based on a daily intake of 2,000 calories. For potassium, aim for foods with a %DV of 5% or less per serving if you're on a low potassium diet.

4. **Ingredients List:** Check the ingredients list for additives and preservatives, as some of these can contain potassium-based compounds.

Remember that food labels are your best friend when it comes to managing your potassium intake.

They provide essential information to help you make informed choices about what you eat.

Cooking Methods and Potassium:

The way you prepare and cook your food can significantly affect its potassium content. Here's how various cooking methods can impact potassium levels:

1. **Boiling:** Boiling vegetables can lead to the loss of potassium as it leaches into the cooking water. To reduce potassium content, you can discard the cooking water or

use it in recipes where the potassium isn't a concern.

2. **Steaming:** Steaming is a gentle cooking method that helps retain potassium in foods. It's an excellent option for those on a low potassium diet.

3. **Microwaving:** Microwaving also helps preserve potassium content, making it a suitable method for low potassium diets.

4. **Roasting and Baking:** These methods don't cause significant potassium loss and can add flavor to your dishes.

5. **Grilling:** Grilling can slightly reduce potassium levels, but it's generally a safe cooking method for those on a low potassium diet.

6. **Frying:** Frying, especially deep frying, can increase potassium content in certain foods due to oil absorption. It's best to avoid this method if you're trying to limit potassium.

7. **Canning and Preserved Foods:** Canned vegetables and fruits may have higher potassium levels due to processing. When possible,

opt for fresh or frozen alternatives.

8. **Fresh vs. Canned:** When choosing fruits and vegetables, fresh options are generally lower in potassium compared to canned or processed varieties.

It's essential to adapt your cooking methods to align with your dietary needs. For instance, if you're preparing a meal that includes high-potassium ingredients, using cooking methods that minimize potassium loss can help you stay within your recommended limits.

In conclusion, Chapter 2 has provided a comprehensive understanding of potassium sources, from common foods that are naturally high in potassium to the importance of reading food labels to deciphering potassium content. We've also explored how different cooking methods can impact the potassium levels in your meals. Armed with this knowledge, you're better equipped to make informed dietary choices as you embark on your journey to successfully follow a low potassium diet. The subsequent chapters will delve even deeper into the practical aspects of managing your potassium intake and maintaining a healthy, balanced diet tailored to your specific needs.

CHAPTER 3

Health Conditions Requiring a Low Potassium Diet

In this chapter, we'll delve into the various health conditions that may necessitate a low potassium diet. While potassium is a vital nutrient for most individuals, certain medical conditions can disrupt the body's potassium balance, leading to potential health risks. Understanding these conditions is crucial for anyone considering or advised to follow a low potassium diet.

1. Chronic Kidney Disease (CKD): Chronic Kidney Disease is perhaps the most common condition that requires a low potassium diet. The kidneys play a pivotal role in maintaining potassium balance in the body. When they function correctly, excess potassium is excreted through urine. However, in CKD, the kidneys progressively lose their ability to filter potassium effectively, resulting in elevated levels of potassium in the blood, a condition known as hyperkalemia.

Hyperkalemia can have severe consequences. High potassium levels can disrupt the normal electrical activity of the heart, leading to irregular heart rhythms and even cardiac arrest. Therefore, individuals with CKD, especially those in advanced stages, are often advised to limit their potassium intake.

2. Kidney Dialysis: For individuals with end-stage kidney disease, dialysis is a life-saving treatment that helps filter waste and excess substances from the blood, including potassium. However, even with dialysis, potassium can build up between sessions, so individuals on dialysis are also typically advised to follow a low potassium diet.

Dietary potassium restrictions in dialysis patients are usually less stringent than those for individuals with CKD who are not on dialysis. Still, it's essential for dialysis patients to manage their potassium intake to prevent complications.

3. Cardiovascular Conditions: Certain heart conditions, particularly those affecting the heart's electrical conduction system, can be exacerbated by high potassium levels. These conditions include:

- **Arrhythmias:** Abnormal heart rhythms can be triggered by high potassium levels. Individuals with arrhythmias may need to limit potassium intake to help manage their condition.
- **Heart Failure:** Some individuals with heart failure may experience an increased risk of hyperkalemia, as the heart's reduced pumping efficiency can affect potassium balance.

- **Medications:** Some medications used to treat heart conditions, like angiotensin-converting enzyme (ACE) inhibitors and angiotensin receptor blockers (ARBs), can increase potassium levels in the blood. Individuals on these medications may need to monitor their potassium intake carefully.

4. **Medications:** Aside from heart medications, various drugs can affect potassium levels. Potassium-sparing diuretics, for example, are a type of medication

that can increase potassium retention in the body, potentially leading to hyperkalemia. In such cases, healthcare providers may recommend a low potassium diet to help offset the medication's effects.

5. Gastrointestinal Disorders: Certain gastrointestinal conditions can disrupt the body's ability to regulate potassium. For example, chronic diarrhea can lead to potassium depletion, while chronic constipation can cause potassium buildup. Individuals with these conditions may need dietary adjustments to manage their potassium levels effectively.

6. Adrenal Gland Disorders:

The adrenal glands produce hormones that regulate potassium levels among other functions. Disorders of the adrenal glands, such as Addison's disease, can affect potassium balance. Depending on the severity of the condition, individuals may require a low potassium diet as part of their treatment plan.

7. Other Medical Conditions:

Various other medical conditions, such as systemic lupus erythematosus (SLE), amyloidosis, and some rare genetic disorders, can impact potassium levels. For individuals with these conditions, healthcare providers will assess potassium balance and recommend dietary modifications as needed.

It's important to emphasize that the need for a low potassium diet should be determined by a healthcare provider based on individual health assessments and laboratory tests. Self-imposing potassium restrictions without medical guidance can lead to nutrient imbalances and may not be necessary.

Assessment and Monitoring:
Individuals with health conditions that may require a low potassium diet will undergo regular assessments and monitoring. This typically involves:

- **Blood Tests:** Regular blood tests, including serum potassium levels, are conducted to assess potassium balance and make necessary dietary adjustments.

- **Dietary Evaluation:** A registered dietitian or nutritionist often plays a key role in assessing an individual's dietary habits and crafting a personalized low potassium diet plan.

- **Medication Management:** If medications are contributing to potassium imbalances, healthcare providers may adjust dosages or prescribe alternative medications.

Balancing Nutrient Intake: While managing potassium intake is crucial for those on a low potassium diet, it's equally important to ensure a balanced intake of other essential nutrients. A well-planned diet can help prevent nutrient deficiencies. This might involve:

- **Monitoring Sodium:** Reducing sodium (salt) intake is often necessary for individuals with kidney disease and certain heart conditions. Managing sodium can help control blood pressure and fluid balance.
- **Protein Intake:** Adequate protein intake is essential for maintaining muscle mass and overall health. A dietitian can help determine

the right amount of protein for your specific needs.

- **Calcium and Phosphorus:** Individuals with kidney disease may also need to manage their calcium and phosphorus intake to prevent complications like bone disease.

- **Fluid Intake:** For some individuals, particularly those on dialysis, monitoring fluid intake is crucial to prevent fluid overload.

In Conclusion: Chapter 3 has explored various health conditions that may necessitate a low potassium diet. It's important to remember that a low potassium diet should always be guided by a healthcare provider and tailored to the individual's specific needs. Regular monitoring, dietary adjustments, and medication management are essential components of successfully managing potassium balance in the context of these health conditions. In the next chapters, we will delve further into the practical aspects of creating a balanced low potassium diet and living well while adhering to these dietary restrictions.

CHAPTER 4

Creating a Balanced Low Potassium Diet

In Chapter 4, we'll delve into the practical aspects of creating and maintaining a balanced low potassium diet. While it's essential to limit potassium intake for specific health conditions, it's equally crucial to ensure that your diet remains balanced and nutritionally adequate. This chapter will guide you through the process of planning your meals, making smart food choices, and providing you with sample meal plans and recipes to get you started.

Understanding Dietary Restrictions: The first step in creating a balanced low potassium diet is understanding your specific dietary restrictions. Your healthcare provider or a registered dietitian will provide guidance on your recommended daily potassium intake, which will depend on the severity of your condition. This intake will be tailored to your unique needs, taking into consideration factors like your age, sex, weight, and the stage of your health condition.

It's important to note that the level of potassium restriction can vary significantly among individuals. Some may need to limit potassium more severely than others, and the duration of dietary restrictions can also vary. Therefore, it's crucial to follow your healthcare provider's recommendations closely.

Meal Planning: Once you understand your dietary restrictions, it's time to embark on meal planning. Planning your meals in advance can help you stay within your potassium limits while ensuring you receive adequate nutrition.

Balanced Meals: A balanced low potassium diet includes a variety of foods from different food groups. Here's how to structure your meals:

1. **Protein:** Include a source of lean protein in each meal. Options may include poultry, fish, lean cuts of beef or pork (in moderation), tofu, legumes, and low-potassium dairy products.

2. **Carbohydrates:** Choose complex carbohydrates like

whole grains (e.g., brown rice, quinoa, whole wheat pasta), as they tend to be lower in potassium than refined grains.

3. **Vegetables:** While some vegetables are high in potassium, others are lower and can be included in your diet. Be sure to cook them using low-potassium methods, such as steaming or microwaving.

4. **Fruits:** Limit high-potassium fruits, but you can enjoy small servings of low-potassium options, such as apples, berries, and grapes.

5. **Fats:** Include healthy fats like olive oil, avocados (in moderation), and nuts (in moderation) to round out your meals.

6. **Dairy:** If your potassium restrictions allow, choose low-potassium dairy products like skim milk or lactose-free options. Otherwise, consider non-dairy alternatives like almond or rice milk.

Portion Control: Controlling portion sizes is crucial when following a low potassium diet. Smaller portions of high-potassium foods can be included in your meals, but you must adhere to your recommended serving sizes to stay within your potassium limits.

Sample Meal Plans: Let's explore some sample meal plans to give you a better idea of what a balanced low potassium diet might look like:

Meal Plan 1:

- Breakfast: Scrambled eggs with spinach and tomatoes (cooked using low-potassium methods), whole wheat toast, and a small serving of berries.

- Snack: Greek yogurt (if potassium restrictions allow).

- Lunch: Grilled chicken breast, brown rice, and steamed broccoli.

- Snack: Carrot sticks with hummus.

- Dinner: Baked salmon (in moderation), quinoa, and sautéed zucchini (cooked using low-potassium methods).

- Dessert (if potassium restrictions allow): A small piece of angel food cake.

Meal Plan 2 (Vegetarian):

- Breakfast: Oatmeal made with water, topped with sliced apples (in moderation) and a sprinkle of cinnamon.
- Snack: Almonds (in moderation).
- Lunch: Lentil soup, a side salad with low-potassium vegetables, and a whole wheat roll.
- Snack: Sliced cucumber with a drizzle of olive oil and vinegar.
- Dinner: Tofu stir-fry with mixed vegetables (low-

potassium choices), served over brown rice.

- Dessert (if potassium restrictions allow): A small serving of sorbet.

These sample meal plans offer a starting point for creating your own low potassium meals. Remember to consult with a registered dietitian or healthcare provider to ensure that these plans align with your specific dietary restrictions.

Recipe Modifications: Adapting recipes to meet your low potassium needs is a valuable skill.

Here are some tips for modifying recipes:

1. **Substitute High-Potassium Ingredients:** Identify high-potassium ingredients in recipes and replace them with lower-potassium alternatives. For instance, replace regular potatoes with sweet potatoes or cauliflower.

2. **Adjust Seasonings:** Experiment with low-potassium herbs and seasonings to add flavor to your dishes. Avoid high-potassium salt substitutes.

3. **Limit Dairy:** If you need to restrict dairy, explore non-dairy alternatives like almond milk or coconut milk (check for potassium content).

4. **Use Low-Potassium Cooking Methods:** Opt for cooking methods like steaming, microwaving, and roasting to minimize potassium loss.

Staying Hydrated: Proper hydration is essential for overall health. However, individuals with kidney disease and certain health conditions may need to monitor their fluid intake. Your healthcare provider will provide guidance on your fluid restrictions if necessary.

Working with a Dietitian: For many individuals on a low potassium diet, working with a registered dietitian is highly beneficial. Dietitians can create personalized meal plans, help you navigate food choices, and ensure that you receive adequate nutrition while adhering to potassium restrictions. They can also provide ongoing support and monitor your progress.

Conclusion: Chapter 4 has explored the practical aspects of creating a balanced low potassium diet. By understanding your dietary restrictions, planning balanced meals, controlling portion sizes, and making smart food choices, you can effectively manage your potassium intake while maintaining overall health. Sample meal plans and recipe modifications provide you with practical tools to get started on your journey to a healthier, balanced diet tailored to your specific needs. Remember that consulting with a healthcare provider or registered dietitian is essential for personalized guidance and support as you navigate your low potassium diet.

CHAPTER 5

Dining Out and Low Potassium Diet

In Chapter 5, we'll navigate the often challenging terrain of dining out while adhering to a low potassium diet. While managing your potassium intake at home is relatively straightforward, eating out at restaurants requires careful planning and communication. This chapter will provide you with strategies, tips, and practical advice to help you enjoy restaurant meals while staying within your dietary restrictions.

Why Dining Out Can Be Tricky:

Eating out presents unique challenges for individuals on a low potassium diet for several reasons:

1. **Limited Control:** Unlike cooking at home, you have limited control over the ingredients and preparation methods used in restaurant dishes.

2. **Hidden Potassium:** Some high-potassium ingredients might be used sparingly but

still add up in restaurant dishes. These ingredients can be hard to identify by taste alone.

3. **Menu Variety:** Restaurant menus often feature a wide range of dishes, making it necessary to navigate through various options to find suitable low potassium choices.

4. **Social Pressure:** Dining out is often a social activity, and you may feel pressured to order dishes that don't align with your dietary restrictions.

Despite these challenges, dining out can still be an enjoyable experience with some careful planning and assertive communication.

Strategies for Dining Out on a Low Potassium Diet:

1. **Choose the Right Restaurant:**
   - Research restaurants in advance: Look for eateries that offer a variety of dishes and are known for accommodating special dietary requests.

- Call ahead: Contact the restaurant ahead of time to inquire about their menu options and willingness to accommodate dietary restrictions.

2. **Review the Menu Carefully:**

- Take your time: Don't feel rushed. Review the menu carefully and look for dishes that are likely to be lower in potassium.

- Avoid buzzwords: Be cautious of menu items described as "creamy," "smothered," or "au gratin," as these often indicate higher potassium content.

3. **Customize Your Order:**

   - Don't hesitate to ask: Politely ask your server to customize your meal. Request modifications like omitting high-potassium ingredients or asking for specific cooking methods.

   - Substitutions: Inquire if the restaurant can substitute high-potassium sides with lower-potassium options. For example, swap out mashed potatoes for a baked sweet potato.

4. **Communicate Clearly:**

   o Be specific: Clearly communicate your dietary restrictions to your server. Explain that you need to limit potassium intake and ask if they can accommodate your needs.

   o Ask questions: Don't hesitate to ask questions about the

ingredients or preparation methods used in dishes you're interested in.

5. **Be Mindful of Hidden Potassium:**

- o Sauces and dressings: High-potassium sauces and dressings can sneak into your meal. Request sauces on the side or inquire about low-potassium alternatives.

- o Seasonings: Be aware that restaurant chefs may use seasonings that contain potassium. Ask if they can use alternatives or limit the use of high-potassium seasonings.

6. **Portion Control:**

   - Restaurant portions can be quite generous. Consider sharing a dish with a dining companion or ask for a to-go box to take leftovers home.

7. **Plan Your Beverages:**

   - Be cautious with beverages: Some beverages like orange juice and tomato juice are high in potassium.

Opt for low-potassium options like water, unsweetened tea, or lemonade.

8. **Dessert Decisions:**

   - Desserts can be a challenge for individuals on a low potassium diet. Consider ordering a dessert that aligns with your dietary restrictions or enjoy a small serving of a low-potassium fruit if it's available.

Cuisine-Specific Tips:

Different types of cuisine may present varying challenges and opportunities for individuals on a low potassium diet. Here are some cuisine-specific tips:

- **Italian:** Italian cuisine often features tomato-based sauces and cheese, both of which can be high in potassium. Look for pasta dishes with non-tomato sauces like pesto or oil-based options. Opt for lower-potassium cheeses like mozzarella.

- **Mexican:** Mexican dishes may contain high-potassium

ingredients like avocados, beans, and tomatoes. Consider ordering fajitas with lean protein and requesting guacamole and salsa on the side. Corn tortillas are generally lower in potassium than flour tortillas.

- **Asian:** Asian cuisine offers a variety of options. Stir-fries with plenty of vegetables can be a good choice, but ask for sauces to be served on the side. Be cautious with soy sauce, which is high in potassium, and use it sparingly or inquire about low-sodium alternatives.

- **Steakhouses:** Steak can be a low-potassium choice if prepared simply. Request lean cuts of meat, like sirloin, and ask for them to be grilled without high-potassium seasonings. Choose side dishes carefully, opting for vegetables prepared with low-potassium methods.

Navigating Fast Food:

While fast food is often associated with convenience and speed, it can also pose challenges for those on a low potassium diet due to the frequent use of high-potassium ingredients. However, there are still options available:

- **Grilled chicken:** Many fast-food restaurants offer grilled chicken sandwiches. Order them without sauces or seasonings high in potassium.
- **Salads:** Choose salads with grilled chicken or other lean protein sources. Request dressing on the side and be cautious of high-potassium toppings like tomatoes and avocados.

- **Sides:** Look for side options like plain baked potatoes or steamed vegetables (if available) and ask for them without high-potassium toppings.

- **Beverages:** Opt for low-potassium beverages like water, diet soda, or unsweetened iced tea.

Dealing with Social Situations:

Eating out often involves social gatherings, and it's natural to feel some social pressure to conform to group choices. Here are some tips for handling these situations:

- **Communicate in advance:** Let your friends or dining companions know about your dietary restrictions in advance so they can choose a restaurant that accommodates your needs.

- **Be assertive, not apologetic:** When ordering, be clear and assertive about your dietary restrictions without feeling the need to apologize. Your health is a top priority.

- **Focus on the company:** Remember that the primary purpose of dining out is to enjoy the company of friends or loved ones. While food is important, it's not the sole focus of the gathering.

Conclusion: Chapter 5 has explored strategies and practical tips for dining out while adhering to a low potassium diet. Eating out can be enjoyable and manageable with careful planning, clear communication with restaurant staff, and an understanding of your dietary restrictions. Remember that flexibility and assertiveness are your allies when navigating restaurant menus, and you can still savor the dining experience while prioritizing your health.

CHAPTER 6

Living Well on a Low Potassium Diet

In Chapter 6, we'll focus on the broader aspects of living well while adhering to a low potassium diet. Beyond meal planning and dining out, this chapter delves into essential lifestyle considerations, emotional well-being, and strategies to maintain a positive and fulfilling life despite dietary restrictions.

Embracing a Positive Mindset:

Living with dietary restrictions, such as a low potassium diet, can be challenging, but maintaining a positive mindset is crucial for your overall well-being. Here are some strategies to help you cultivate a positive outlook:

1. **Education:** Understanding the reasons behind your dietary restrictions can empower you. Knowledge about your condition and the importance of your diet can reduce anxiety and uncertainty.

2. **Support System:** Connect with friends, family, or

support groups who understand your dietary needs. Sharing your challenges and successes can be uplifting.

3. **Focus on What You Can Eat:** Instead of dwelling on foods you should avoid, concentrate on the delicious and nutritious options that are still available to you. Explore new recipes and ingredients to make your meals exciting.

4. **Mindful Eating:** Savor your meals by eating slowly, appreciating flavors, and enjoying the sensory

experience of dining. This can enhance your satisfaction with low-potassium foods.

5. **Celebrate Small Wins:** Acknowledge and celebrate your achievements, whether it's sticking to your dietary plan for a week or trying a new low-potassium recipe.

Staying Active:

Physical activity plays a significant role in maintaining overall health, even while on a low potassium diet. Here's how to incorporate exercise into your lifestyle:

1. **Consult Your Healthcare Provider:** Before starting any new exercise routine, consult your healthcare provider to ensure it's safe for your specific health condition.

2. **Choose Activities You Enjoy:** Engaging in activities you like increases the likelihood that you'll stick with them. Whether it's walking, swimming, yoga, or gardening, find activities that bring you joy.

3. **Adapt Your Routine:** If your health condition affects your energy levels or

mobility, consider adapted exercise options. Chair exercises or physical therapy exercises can be effective and safe.

4. **Stay Hydrated:** Proper hydration is essential, especially when you're physically active. Be mindful of your fluid restrictions if you have them, and adjust your water intake accordingly.

5. **Listen to Your Body:** Pay attention to how your body responds to exercise. If you experience discomfort or pain, modify your routine or

consult your healthcare provider.

Managing Stress:

Chronic health conditions and dietary restrictions can sometimes lead to stress and anxiety. Here are strategies to help manage stress effectively:

1. **Relaxation Techniques:** Practice relaxation techniques such as deep breathing, meditation, or progressive muscle relaxation to reduce stress.

2. **Time Management:** Organize your daily activities

and priorities to reduce stressors. Effective time management can help you achieve a sense of control.

3. **Seek Support:** Share your feelings with friends, family, or a therapist. Emotional support is essential for managing stress.

4. **Engage in Stress-Relief Activities:** Pursue hobbies or activities that help you relax and unwind, whether it's reading, listening to music, or spending time in nature.

5. **Maintain a Balanced Lifestyle:** Strive for a

balanced life that includes adequate rest, physical activity, social interactions, and relaxation.

Staying Socially Active:

Social connections are vital for emotional well-being. Don't let dietary restrictions isolate you. Here's how to stay socially active:

1. **Communicate Your Needs:** When planning social events or dining with friends and family, communicate your dietary restrictions and preferences. Most people will be

understanding and accommodating.

2. **Host Gatherings:** Consider hosting gatherings or potlucks where you can prepare low-potassium dishes that everyone can enjoy. This puts you in control of the menu.

3. **Explore New Experiences:** Participate in social activities that don't revolve around food, such as movie nights, game nights, or outdoor adventures.

4. **Join Support Groups:** Look for local or online support groups for

individuals with similar dietary restrictions. Connecting with others who understand your challenges can be comforting.

5. **Volunteer or Give Back:** Engaging in volunteer work or community activities not only strengthens social connections but also provides a sense of purpose.

Adapting to Special Occasions:

Special occasions and holidays can be tricky to navigate on a low potassium diet, but they don't have to be overwhelming. Here are strategies to help you enjoy these times:

1. **Plan in Advance:** Plan your meals for special occasions carefully. You can work with a dietitian to create a special menu or choose restaurants that offer low-potassium options.

2. **Communicate Your Needs:** Let hosts or event organizers know about your dietary restrictions in advance. They may be willing to make accommodations.

3. **Contribute to the Meal:**
Offer to bring a dish that fits
within your dietary
guidelines. This ensures you
have at least one safe option
to enjoy.

4. **Practice Portion
Control:** During special
occasions, it's easy to
overindulge. Focus on small
portions of your favorite
dishes to stay within your
potassium limits.

5. **Enjoy Non-Food
Traditions:** Celebrations
aren't solely about the food.
Participate in non-food
traditions, such as games,

music, or storytelling, to create lasting memories.

Traveling with Dietary Restrictions:

Traveling can present unique challenges for those on a low potassium diet. However, with proper planning, you can still enjoy safe and memorable trips:

1. **Research Your Destination:** Before traveling, research the local cuisine and available dining options. Look for restaurants that offer low-potassium choices.

2. **Pack Smart:** Consider packing non-perishable, low-potassium snacks for the journey, like nuts (if potassium restrictions allow), dried fruits (in moderation), or rice cakes.

3. **Communicate with Accommodations:** If you're staying in a hotel, contact them in advance to inquire about meal options that align with your dietary needs.

4. **Carry Documentation:** Have a medical alert card or note from your healthcare provider that explains your

dietary restrictions in case of emergency or language barriers.

5. **Stay Hydrated:** Maintain proper hydration, especially if you're traveling to a warm climate. Be mindful of your fluid restrictions if applicable.

Dining Out While Traveling:

Eating out during travel is a common activity, and it's essential to continue following your dietary restrictions. Here are tips for dining out while traveling:

1. **Use Translation Apps:** If you're traveling to a foreign country with a language barrier, consider using translation apps to communicate your dietary needs to restaurant staff.

2. **Research Local Cuisine:** Learn about the typical dishes and ingredients of the region you're visiting. This knowledge can help you make informed menu choices.

3. **Consult Online Reviews:** Check online reviews and forums for recommendations on

restaurants that cater to dietary restrictions in your travel destination.

4. **Pack Snacks:** Carry low-potassium snacks with you while sightseeing to curb hunger between meals and prevent the temptation to eat high-potassium street foods.

Conclusion:

Chapter 6 has explored essential aspects of living well on a low potassium diet. Embracing a positive mindset, staying physically active, managing stress, maintaining social connections, adapting to special occasions, and traveling with dietary restrictions are all part of the journey to living a fulfilling and healthy life despite the challenges posed by dietary restrictions. Remember that flexibility, communication, and self-care are key elements in maintaining overall well-being while adhering to a low potassium diet.

CHAPTER 7

Long-Term Success and Resources for Your Low Potassium Diet

In the final chapter of our guide, we'll delve into the strategies and resources for achieving long-term success while following a low potassium diet. We'll explore how to maintain motivation, monitor your progress, and find ongoing support. Additionally, we'll discuss valuable resources and tools that can aid you on your journey.

Maintaining Motivation:

Sustaining motivation over the long term is essential for successfully managing a low potassium diet. Here are some strategies to help you stay motivated:

1. **Set Realistic Goals:** Establish achievable short-term and long-term goals related to your dietary restrictions. Celebrate your achievements along the way.

2. **Visualize Success:** Imagine the benefits of maintaining a low potassium diet. Visualizing improved health and well-being can be a powerful motivator.

3. **Stay Informed:** Keep up-to-date with the latest

research and developments related to your health condition. Understanding the positive impact of your diet can be motivating.

4. **Track Your Progress:** Maintain a record of your dietary choices, lab results, and how you feel. Seeing tangible improvements can reinforce your commitment.

5. **Seek Support:** Share your goals with friends, family, or a support group. Having a support system can provide encouragement when motivation wanes.

6. **Reward Yourself:** Treat yourself when you achieve milestones. Rewards can be as simple as enjoying a favorite activity or indulging in a small, non-dietary pleasure.

Ongoing Monitoring:

Continual monitoring of your low potassium diet is crucial for adapting to changing needs and ensuring that you remain on the right track. Here's how to approach ongoing monitoring:

1. **Regular Check-Ups:** Schedule regular

appointments with your healthcare provider to assess your health status, including potassium levels. These visits allow for adjustments to your dietary plan as needed.

2. **Food Journaling:** Maintain a food diary to keep track of your meals, snacks, and any symptoms or changes in health. This journal can be helpful during healthcare appointments.

3. **Lab Tests:** Follow your healthcare provider's recommendations for regular blood tests to

monitor potassium levels and other relevant markers.

4. **Medication Review:** If you're taking medications that affect potassium balance, ensure that your healthcare provider reviews and adjusts your prescriptions as necessary.

5. **Dietitian Consultations:** Continue to work with a registered dietitian to fine-tune your meal plans and receive ongoing guidance.

6. **Self-Assessment:** Periodically assess how well you're adhering to your dietary restrictions and

address any areas where you might be struggling.

Finding Ongoing Support:

Support is essential for long-term success on a low potassium diet. Here are ways to find and maintain support throughout your journey:

1. **Online Communities:** Explore online forums and support groups dedicated to individuals with dietary restrictions. These communities provide a platform for sharing experiences and tips.

2. **Local Support Groups:**
Look for local support
groups or health
organizations that offer in-
person meetings or events
related to your health
condition and diet.

3. **Family and Friends:** Lean
on the support of your loved
ones. Educate them about
your dietary restrictions so
they can better understand
and assist you.

4. **Professional Guidance:**
Continue to work with
healthcare professionals,
including your primary care
physician, nephrologist,

dietitian, and any other specialists relevant to your health condition.

5. **Mental Health Support:** If you're experiencing emotional challenges related to your diet, consider seeking support from a therapist or counselor.

Valuable Resources and Tools:

Several resources and tools are available to help you navigate your low potassium diet effectively. Here are some valuable ones to consider:

1. **Registered Dietitians:** Dietitians are an invaluable resource for personalized guidance, meal planning, and ongoing support. Consult with a dietitian regularly.

2. **Cookbooks and Recipes:** Many cookbooks and websites offer low-potassium recipes and meal ideas. These resources can inspire creativity in the kitchen.

3. **Mobile Apps:** Some mobile apps are designed to help individuals track their potassium intake and make informed food choices.

4. **Food Label Guides:** Familiarize yourself with guides that explain how to read food labels, including potassium content. This knowledge empowers you to make informed choices at the grocery store.

5. **Health Apps and Wearables:** Health apps and wearable devices can assist with tracking diet, exercise, and overall health metrics.

6. **Educational Materials:** Seek out educational materials from reputable health organizations and

websites that provide in-depth information about your health condition and dietary restrictions.

7. **Cooking Classes:** Consider enrolling in cooking classes focused on low-potassium cooking. These classes can enhance your culinary skills and introduce you to new ingredients.

Adapting Over Time:

As you continue your journey on a low potassium diet, remember that dietary needs can change over time. Be open to adjustments and consult with your healthcare team as needed. Here are common scenarios where adaptations may be necessary:

1. **Health Condition Progression:** If your health condition progresses, your dietary restrictions may become more stringent. Your healthcare provider and dietitian will guide you through these changes.

2. **Medication Changes:** If you start or stop medications that affect potassium balance, your dietary requirements may need adjustment.

3. **Aging:** Nutritional needs can change as you age. Be prepared for potential shifts in your dietary recommendations.

4. **Life Events:** Major life events such as pregnancy, surgery, or illness can impact your dietary needs. Communicate with your healthcare provider during such times.

5. **New Research:** Stay informed about new research and advancements in the field of nutrition and your specific health condition. Your healthcare

provider may adjust your diet based on the latest findings.

In Conclusion:

Chapter 7 emphasizes the importance of long-term success on a low potassium diet. By maintaining motivation, continually monitoring your progress, finding ongoing support, and utilizing valuable resources and tools, you can effectively manage your dietary restrictions and lead a fulfilling and healthy life. Remember that flexibility and adaptation are key to addressing changing needs over time. With the right strategies and support in place, you can successfully navigate the challenges of a low potassium diet while prioritizing your health and well-being.

CONCLUSION

In conclusion, our comprehensive guide has provided a thorough exploration of the principles and practicalities of a low potassium diet. We've journeyed through seven chapters, each addressing vital aspects of managing this dietary restriction. Let's recap the key takeaways from each chapter:

Chapter 1: We began by understanding the fundamentals of potassium, its importance, and how it's managed in the body. This foundational knowledge is crucial for grasping why a low potassium diet might be necessary.

Chapter 2: Building on our understanding, we explored dietary sources of potassium and learned how to identify high-potassium foods. This knowledge is essential for making informed food choices.

Chapter 3: We delved into the various health conditions that may require a low potassium diet, emphasizing that such dietary restrictions should always be guided by a healthcare provider based on individual health assessments.

Chapter 4: Practicality took center stage as we learned how to create balanced low potassium meals, manage portion sizes, and adapt recipes to meet our dietary needs.

Chapter 5: Dining out, a common social activity, was explored in depth. We discussed strategies for making wise food choices in restaurants, regardless of cuisine or occasion.

Chapter 6: The broader aspects of living well on a low potassium diet were addressed, from maintaining a positive mindset and staying active to managing stress and embracing social interactions. We also discussed strategies for adapting to special occasions and traveling with dietary restrictions.

Chapter 7: In our final chapter, we focused on long-term success, monitoring progress, and finding ongoing support. We highlighted valuable resources and tools to aid in the journey and emphasized the importance of adaptation as dietary needs evolve.

Ultimately, successfully managing a low potassium diet is a journey that requires a combination of knowledge, planning, ongoing support, and a positive mindset. By taking the lessons from each chapter to heart and applying them in your daily life, you can effectively navigate the challenges of a low potassium diet while prioritizing your health and well-being. Remember that flexibility and adaptation are your allies on this journey, and with the right strategies and support in place, you can lead a fulfilling and healthy life.